LOW CARB MEALS FOR THE BUSY, RUSHED, IMPATIENT, OR LAZY KITCHEN HATER

How to throw a meal together even when you hate cooking!

DR. KRISTA B. ELLOW, PHARMD., BCACP

Disclaimer

This book is not intended as a substitute for the medical recommendations of physicians or other health-care providers.

Rather, it is intended to offer information to help the reader cooperate with physicians and health professionals in a joint quest for optimum health.

FIRST EDITION

www.stophighsugars.com

DEDICATION

To my father, John Baron, who gave me
endless examples of doing what is right,
despite the cost or popular opinion.

Thanks for showing me the way Dad.

- Krista -

Contents

Note from the Author

Dear busy, rushed, impatient or lazy kitchen hater,

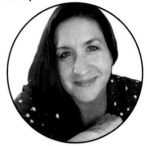

I'm Dr. Krista Ellow and I am the original and the worst of us all. I love the food, but hate the process. I am busy and rushed. I am impatient and sometimes lazy. I will vacuum, pay bills, do laundry, fold laundry, clean up poop, change diapers, mow lawns, pull weeds, drop off kids, pick up kids and even shampoo the carpet... just please don't make me cook dinner!

These sentiments got worse when I realized I needed to make a change for my patients, children and family. I needed to stop stuffing everyone (especially myself) with high carbohydrate food favorites and relearn how to pair food and create meals. This task was daunting at first, but as I began to restructure our meals I realized I already had all the skills I needed.

You see, growing up there was always an abundance of love and support, but not always an abundance of food and proper nutrition. During those times, we did what we could to piece meals together with what we had. Our mother was and still is, the master of this craft. The art of the kitchen scramble; the ability to pull scraps together and form a seemingly planned meal. Where one person saw an empty refrigerator, my mother saw a home cooked meal to fill her family. I guess I was paying attention.

As low-carb became a habit, the effort of pulling food together dropped off the radar. As my diabetes coaching program grew however, it became clear I needed to share what I had learned in order to create lasting success with my clients.

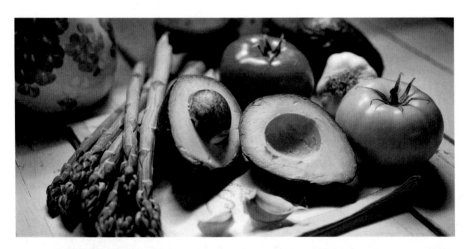

Enter the cookbook for the busy, rushed, impatient and lazy kitchen hater...ME.

This is not your mama's Betty Crocker meal guide. This is about survival. I will not teach you how to cook. I will show you how to look at the food at hand and make something to eat.

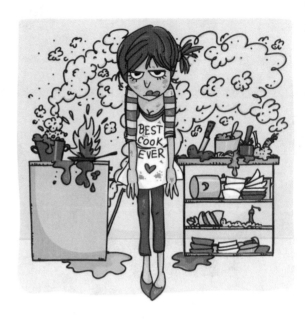

Armed only with the "best low carb food" list, my mother and I created meals one by one. We imagined having each ingredient in the fridge or cupboards and preparing them in a manner we already knew. When you are rushed and busy, you don't whip out the cookbook, you go with what you know. If you don't know how to poach an egg, you are likely not going to start now...or on your busy morning before work. We prepared the food in our head and wrote down how we did it. That simple. That is probably why everything is done in the pan, oven or without any cooking at all. You will also notice that the recipes have very few ingredients. Just looking at a recipe with more than 6 ingredients makes me give up.

The system we used to create these recipes means that the recipes themselves are endless in possibilities, which means you can keep this cookbook going! I hope you will. There are extra pages in the back for just such genius.

You will also notice throughout the book that I take shortcuts like pre-shredded cabbage and beef that is already cut. I even use a cheese stick in my "Cordon-Bleu". I have no time for fancy. Fancy is for restaurants and the White House. I'm busy, rushed and impatient. I need easy. If you feel the same, welcome!

With love and understanding,

Krista

Dr. Krista B. Ellow

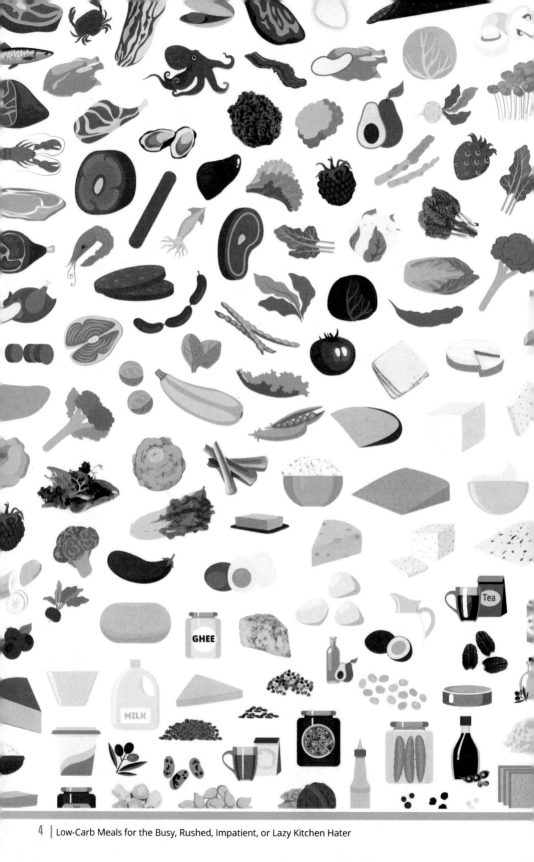

The Secret to Recipe Creation

I am not kidding when I say that I gave my mother only a list of acceptable foods and made her give me recipes on the spot. We didn't even test kitchen most of them, because we knew they would work. We refined them with years of practicing the Kitchen Scramble.

You can do this as well. Below you will find the very list I used to create each meal. A few pointers before we begin.

Salt and pepper is not typically included as an ingredient. I assume you are going to add this as your taste prefers.

The cooking times are also estimated since each dish can vary from prep to prep due to the freshness or thickness of each ingredient. Check more often (every 20 minutes) for recipes that are in the oven.

Ground beef can be substituted for ground turkey or ground pork or even mixed together for variety.

I add chopped onions, celery or peppers to ground beef when cooking to prevent myself from making a beef shaped hockey puck...but it's up to you.

You can season these dishes any way you like. Just like food, we tend to cluster our spices around a dozen or so staples, unless you're a chef or foodie. But you're not because that would mean you enjoy the kitchen. I use garlic salt, onion salt, Italian seasoning, salt, pepper, cinnamon, oregano, parsley and hot sauce.

Loosen up. Recipes were created by trial and error.

Finally, here is how we picked recipes.

We chose a protein source. Paired it with some kind of plant. Topped it with a great tasting condiment, sauce or spice. That's it. Sometimes a single ingredient is great for a snack. Sometimes 3 ingredients created an amazing dinner.

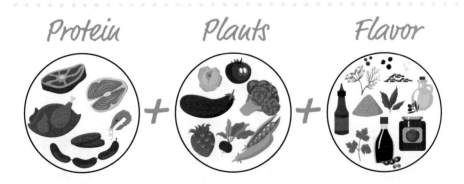

Protein + Plants + Flavor

Meats

Beef

White Fish

Sliced ham

Chicken

Crab

Sliced Pancetta

Game meat

Lobster

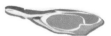
Pastrami

Lamb

Mussels

Prosciutto

Pork

Octopus

Sliced Roast Beef

Veal

Oysters

Sliced Turkey

Bacon

Scallops

Sliced Chorizo

HotDogs

Shrimp

Ground Chorizo

Organ Meats

Squid

Pepperoni

Sausage

Sliced Chicken

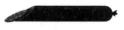
Salami

Fatty Fish

Corned beef

Bologna

Veggies & Berries

 Boston Lettuce

 Mustard Greens

 Radishes

 Cucumbers

 Butter Lettuce

 Spinach

 Broccoli Raab

 Green Beans

 Endive

 Swiss Chard

 Tomatoes

 Okra

 Field Greens

 Turnips

 Zucchini

 Snap Peas

 Iceberg

 Asparagus

 Artichoke

 Bell Peppers

 Turnip Greens

 Avocado

 Broccoli

 Strawberries

 Romaine

 Bok Choy

 Broccolini

 Blackberries

 Watercress

 Celery

 Brussel Sprouts

 Raspberries

 Collard Greens

 Eggplant

 Cabbage

 Blueberries

 Kale

 Mushrooms

 Cauliflower

Dairy & Cold Case

Butter

Gouda

Mozzarella

Ghee (clarified butter)

Muenster

Parmesan

Heavy Cream

Provolone

Pepper Jack

Blue Cheese

Swiss

Cottage Cheese

Brie

Eggs

Greek Yogurt (plain)

Colby

Cheddar Cheese

Ricotta

Cream Cheese

Feta

Sour Cream

Goat

Havarti

Whole Milk

Grocery

 Avocado oil

 Pork Rinds

 Flax Seeds

 Cocoa Butter

 Parmesan Crisps

 Hemp Seeds

 Coconut oil

 Club Soda

 Beef Jerky

 Olive oil

 Coffee

 Coconut Milk

 Canned fish

 Tea

 Artichoke hearts

 Olives

 Brazil Nuts

 Hearts of Palm

 Sauerkraut

 Macadamia Nuts

 Pickles

 Hot Sauce

 Pecans

 Pizza Sauce

 Mayonnaise

 Walnuts

 Tomato Sauce

 Mustard

 Chia Seeds

 Soy Sauce

Spices

Pumpkin Seeds

Remember with all foods to check labels for hidden sugars and sweeteners. Be sure to get uncured or dry cured meats and cheese.

AVOID "CHEESE FOOD".

Since we are lazy and busy, get the deli to cut your meat and cheese.

Go ahead and try making a recipe. Pick a food from each column or just try three columns like many of the recipes have done.

Here, I'll start...

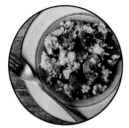

Ground chorizo with eggs on a bed of iceberg lettuce with hot sauce... delicious.

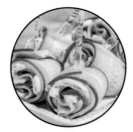

Sliced ham rolled up with swiss cheese and double rolled into cucumber.

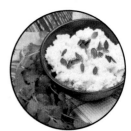

Mixed pumpkins seeds with walnuts over cottage cheese.

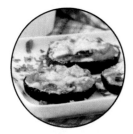

Eggplant slices fried in butter topped with shredded cheddar cheese and pizza sauce.

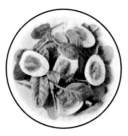

Field greens mixed up with hard-boiled egg slices and mayonnaise.

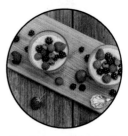

Greek yogurt mixed with fresh strawberries and raspberries.

Literally made them all up as I am writing this book. I might even have doubled those recipes below. Your turn. Pick ingredients you recognize, and know how to prepare, and throw them together! Start with what you already know or you will get frustrated immediately.

Now, you may be tempted to try and incorporate all of the ingredients listed in some form or another, but don't sweat it. Stick with what you like and experiment with the rest. As it stands right now, you only eat about 25 different foods on a regular basis and that is pushing it. There are over 150 food items listed above and many other foods likely deserve to be there, but this is the list most Americans will be familiar with. Chances are good you will not like some of them. To make you feel better, I don't eat veal, lamb or organ meat. I also don't eat artichokes, squid or octopus. I won't even try them. That's ok because there are so many other choices.

A Note on Cooking Oils

Cooking with butter or coconut oil is probably best as these fats are solid at room temperature. Oils and fats that are liquid at room temperature can degrade with the heat of cooking and create unstable free radicals... yes they are real. We should have just stood by butter in the 50s. We had it right.

For my peeps with diabetes, remember you are likely deficient in potassium, despite what your lab test says, due to the insulin resistance. Eat more foods with potassium and magnesium. The top potassium foods are listed below.

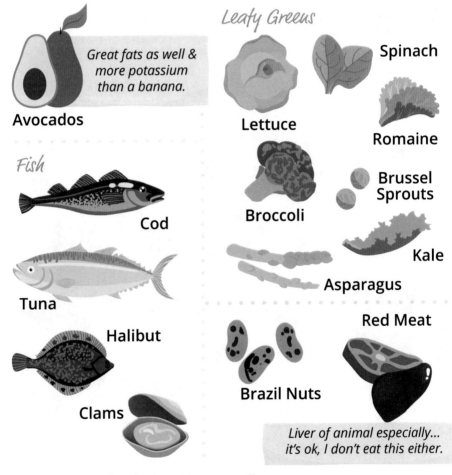

Great fats as well & more potassium than a banana.

Avocados

Leafy Greens

Spinach

Lettuce

Romaine

Fish

Cod

Broccoli

Brussel Sprouts

Kale

Tuna

Asparagus

Halibut

Red Meat

Brazil Nuts

Clams

Liver of animal especially... it's ok, I don't eat this either.

Ok, that is a wrap for the intro, but not a flour or corn wrap... more like a lettuce wrap. Yes, these are the jokes.

Let's start our low-carb options with a chapter in top demand; a chapter that answers the question I get asked daily:
What can I snack on Dr. Ellow?

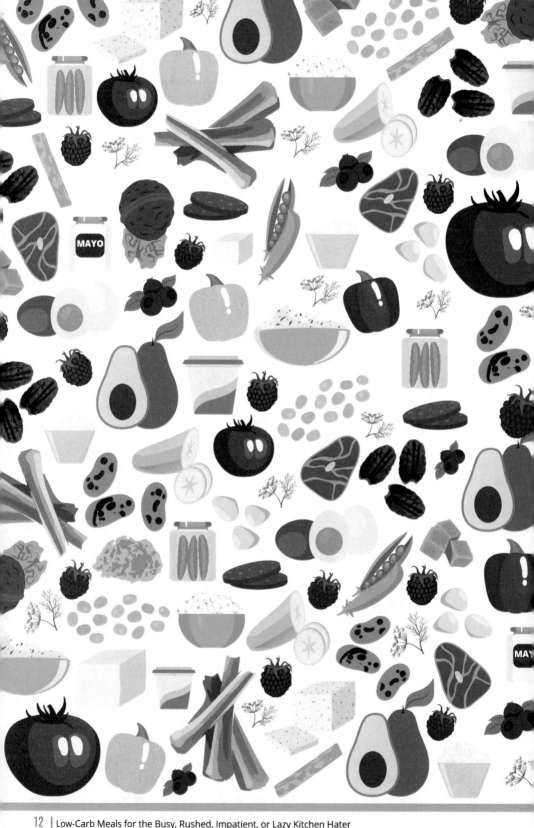

CHAPTER 1
Snacks &
Desk Food

I consider anything I can eat quickly without making a huge mess or putting in much effort a snack. If I made it ahead of time that counts as low effort for snack time. Depending on your appetite and energy use, some of these options can be your lunch as well. Remember, these are just the ones that I made up from my list of foods. Add any that you come up with as well.

Remember that breakfast in the morning is not mandatory. You can do quite well with a cup of coffee or tea with heavy cream, half and half or a spoonful of coconut oil. Breakfast is not the most important meal of the day. Breaking the fast with real food is.

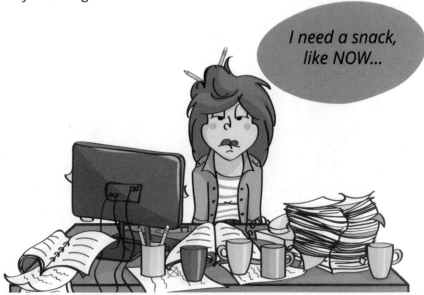

Any Low-Carb Nut

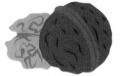

Walnuts

Pecans

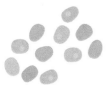

Macadamia

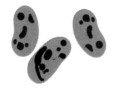

Brazil

Mix nuts together or eat alone.

Keep them in your desk at work.

Be mindful of how much you eat.

They are delicious & the carbs add up quickly.

Celery Sticks

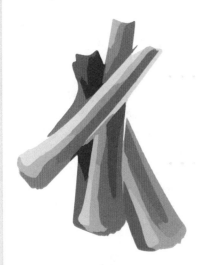

filled with

Cream Cheese

bundled with

Cheese Sticks

dipped in

Creamy Dill Dip

Creamy Dill Dip: equal parts sour cream and mayo mixed with dill weed
Dill weed is strong so add to mix slowly and taste often.

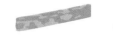

Cheese Sticks + **Pepperoni Slices**

Dry cured pepperoni please.

Check labels as Bread and Butter Pickles are super sweet and have sugar/sweeteners.

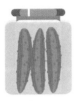 +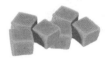

Pickles **Cheese Cubes**

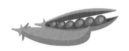 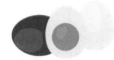

Snap Peas **Hard-Boiled Eggs** **Sweet Peppers**

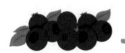 + *or*

Crushed Blueberries **Cottage Cheese** **Ricotta Cheese**

We call this "Bird Poop."

You'll see why...

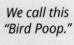

 +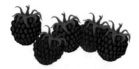

Goat Cheese **Blackberries & Raspberries**

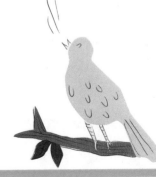

Mini Peppers

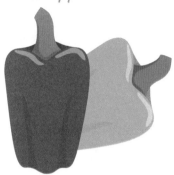

stuffed with

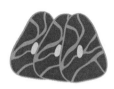
Ham Slices

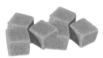
Cheese Cubes

Sliced Tomato

+ **Cream Cheese Sandwich**

or

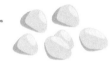
Mozzarella

+
Cucumber

dipped in

Homemade Ranch

I'm sorry...
store bought ranch is just loaded with no-nos.

....

Since you probably don't have this ready ahead of time just mix mayo with sour cream, salt and lemon.

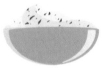

Cucumber Slices

+
Cream Cheese Sandwich

try adding

Tomato Slices

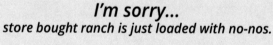

Cheese Crisps

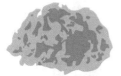

Shredded Cheese

Make ahead of time by placing shredded cheese in cupcake trays and baking until crisp.

Bake at 400 degrees for about 8 minutes.

We figured this out last year by accident and we are hooked.

+

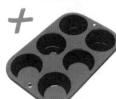

Bake in cupcake tray

=

or

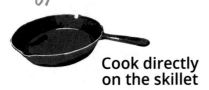

Cook directly on the skillet

try adding

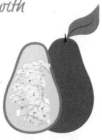

Pepperoni Slices

Same as above, but add a pepperoni slice.

Place a small pile of shredded cheese on a skillet (don't grease).

When the cooked side is crisp flip over and add filling to center (anchovies, olives, breakfast sausage, use your imagination!)

Remove from skillet and enjoy. It's amazing!

Avocado Half Stuffed with

Chicken Salad

Egg Salad

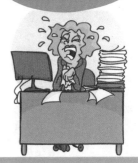

I'm so HANGRY!

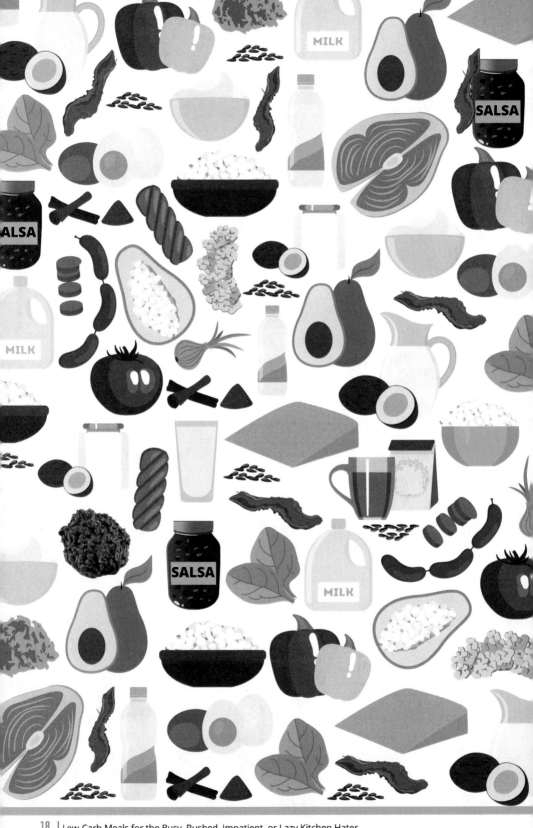

CHAPTER 2
Food We Often Eat at Breakfast

We label certain foods as good for breakfast, but I eat eggs all the time... and so do you very likely. It's a bit weird that egg salad is considered "lunchy" while eggs over easy is strictly "breakfasty". I do not limit myself to such things, and have enjoyed many dinners made of breakfast type food. I encourage you to do the same. Besides, who doesn't enjoy a good Brinner (breakfast at dinner)?

The only times I would encourage you to consider increased thought and planning for food types is when you are breaking a fast and if you are pregnant. Breaking a fast with the wrong food and the wrong amount can cause some serious squirts. And we all know it's important to be vigilant when expecting. Other than that, don't get caught up.

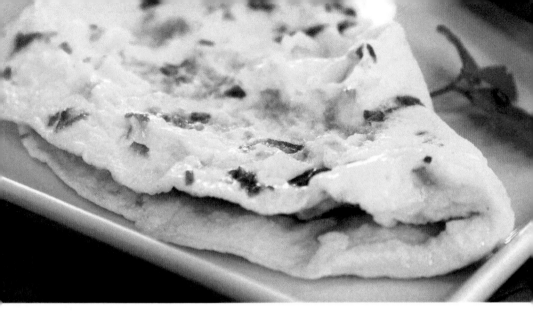

Omelet

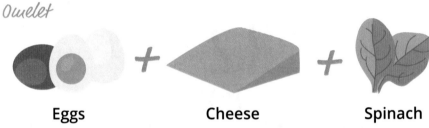

Eggs + **Cheese** + **Spinach**

> *For those that have terrible technique for making omelets,
> I briefed that for you below. If you don't care that it's perfect
> or an omelet, then just mix the ingredients in a bowl and
> pour into a butter fry pan. Stir until cooked.*

1. Beat eggs in small bowl until blended (I often add some filling here as well).

2. Heat butter in non-stick skillet over medium-high heat until hot.

3. Tilt pan to coat bottom.

4. Pour in egg mixture. Mixture should set immediately at edges.

5. GENTLY PUSH cooked portions of egg from edges toward the center with a spatula so that uncooked eggs can reach the hot pan surface.

6. Continue cooking and gently moving cooked portions as needed.

7. When top surface of eggs is thickened and no visible liquid egg remains, place filling on one side of the omelet.

8. Fold omelet in half (no need to flip onto other side since egg is already cooked) and slide onto plate.

Universal Frittata

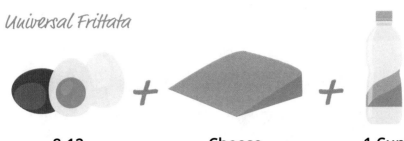

| 8-12 Eggs | Cheese to Taste | 1 Cup Heavy Cream |

Mix in a bowl and pour into greased baking dish.

Bake for 1 hour at 350 or until center is cooked.

You can add any veggies or meat you would like to this recipe, just add before you cook it.

Cut into sections and eat.

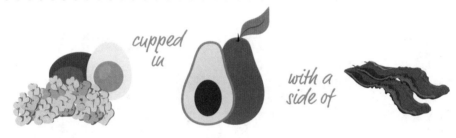

cupped in

with a side of

Eggs
(scrambled is easiest)

Avocado

Bacon

Chia Pudding

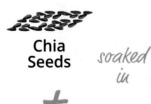

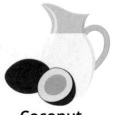

Chia Seeds

soaked in

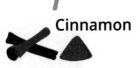

Cinnamon

Coconut Milk

Prep the night before. Usually about 1 tablespoon of chia in 6-8 ounces of milk

Make sure to stir and keep in the fridge until morning.

Bacon, Egg, and Cheese Cups

Line each cup with bacon around the inside.

Mix eggs and cheese in a bowl and pour into each cup... since you have no patience you probably did not check to see how many eggs you needed and will probably run out and have to make a second batch.

Start with as many eggs as there are cups in the cupcake tin and you should be fine.

Add anything else that you would want in an omelet.

Cook in oven at 350 until the eggs and bacon are cooked. Better set a timer.

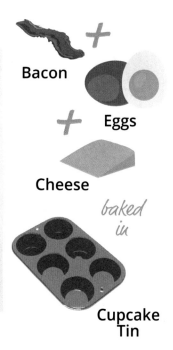

Bacon

+

Eggs

+

Cheese

baked in

Cupcake Tin

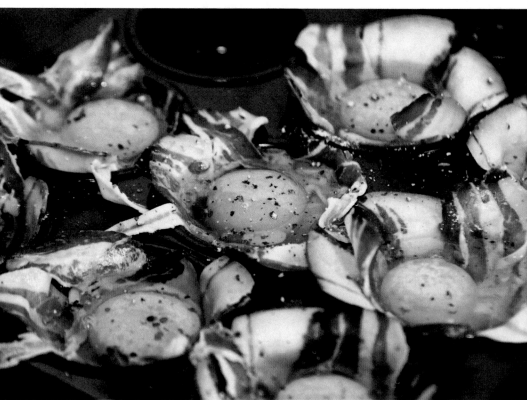

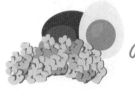

Scrambled Eggs   **Salmon**

Fish is strange to me, but it always works when I put butter in the pan and fry it until cooked.

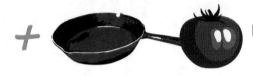

Pan Seared Tomatoes

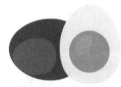 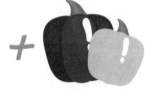 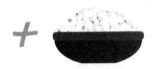

Eggs   **Chopped Bell Peppers**   **Feta Cheese**

Ground Turkey   **Eggs**   **Salsa**

I usually start to brown the ground meat first then add the eggs until cooked. Top with salsa

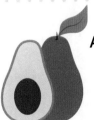

Avocado Half

try adding

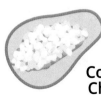

Cottage Cheese

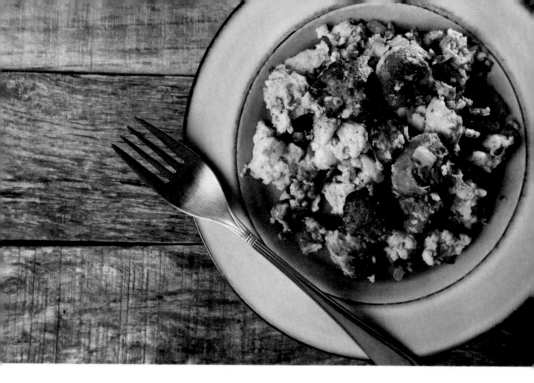

Chorizo & Egg Scramble

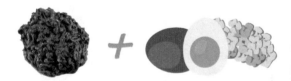

Ground Chorizo + **Eggs**

Typically 4-6 eggs scrambled as the chorizo reduces just a bit more than regular ground meat.

Patties, Peppers, and Onions

Can also buy ground breakfast sausage as well (in the tube).

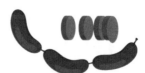

Chopped Sausage Patties

Sautéed Peppers & Onions

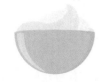 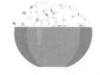 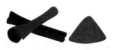

Greek Yogurt + **Cottage Cheese** + **Cinnamon**

*Mix equal parts of Greek yogurt & cottage cheese.
Get full fat, not that ZERO garbage.*

I recommend real food most of the time, but the reality is that you are busy, rushed and impatient. Sometimes we have to compromise.

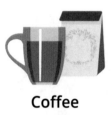

Coffee

A spoonful of Coconut Oil

*OK! But first...
COFFEE!*

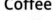 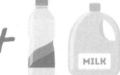

+

Half & Half is just equal parts heavy cream & whole milk.

Half & Half

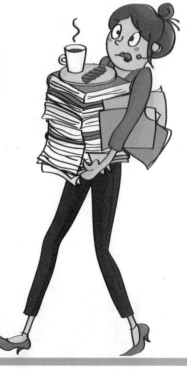

Or grab a keto or low-carb friendly...

Meal Bar *or* **Shake**

My favorite brands are Premier Protein & 310.

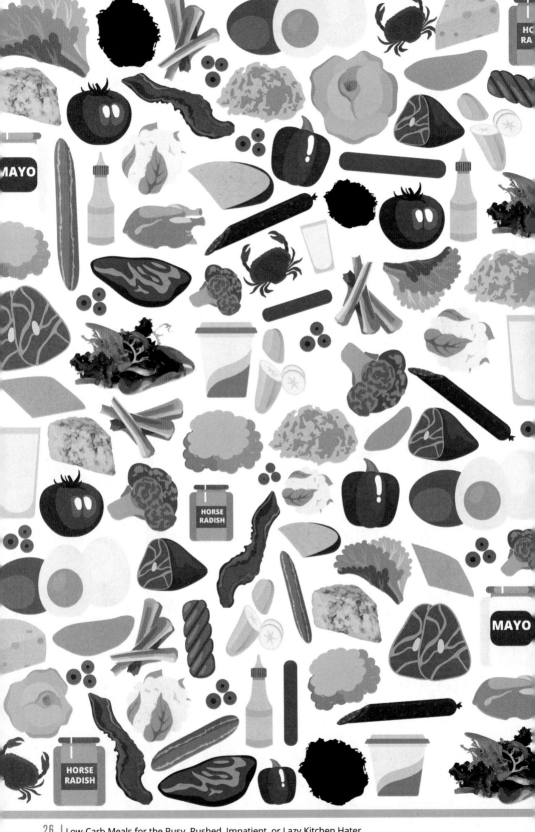

CHAPTER 3
Lunch Meals
to Avoid the Peer Pressure of Ordering Chinese Food at Work

Seriously, the easiest thing you could possibly do for lunch is just make double the dinner the night before. I would even make that serving and put it in the fridge before you eat supper. This ensures you don't accidentally get excited and eat everything. But, if you hate leftovers I wrote out some options below. As a rule I never eat or re-heat fish or seafood at work. Do your co-workers a favor and follow this rule as well.

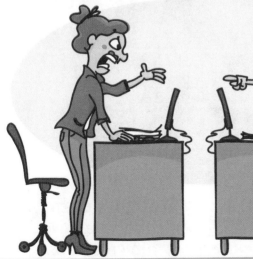
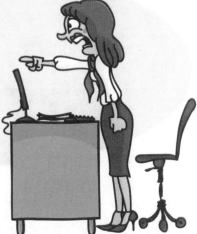

If you have a cafeteria at work and utilize its convenience, head straight to the salad bar and dump greens on your plate. Top those greens with cottage cheese, chicken salad and/or some antipasto. If the entree line has meat and veggies that is great as well; beef with broccoli, chicken with broccoli or pork chops.

Avoid the rice, potatoes, pasta salad and pudding. Don't even make eye contact. Once you have eaten your fill of salad bar, you can go back and stare down the desserts. It's much easier to say no when the hunger is quieted.

Soup is probably not a great idea either. I wish it was, I love soup. The cafeteria soup and most grocery store options have the fake sugar cooked right in. Make soup at home and bring it with you. I give you a recipe in chapter 5.

If you hate brown bagging and like going out, stick with places that have salad type options (Chick-Fil-A, Subway, Chipotle). As my roommate always said, just make good choices.

I can tell you that my lunch is always the meal from the night before in a Rubbermaid container or a bag of frozen veggies I could steam in the microwave with a side of mayo or sour cream... literally.

Like I said, this is not a book on cooking, it's a book on surviving when you are busy and impatient.

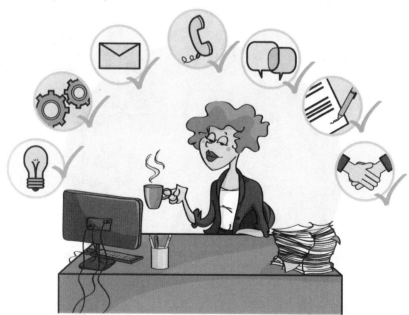

Brown bag your dinner from the night before!
It's easier to get stuff done when you aren't worried
about what you're going to get for lunch.

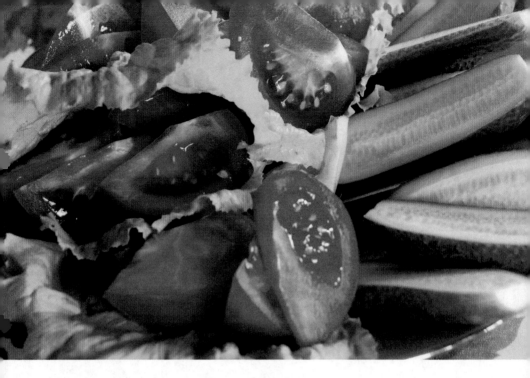

salads

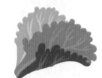

Romaine Lettuce Leaves

topped with

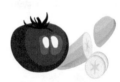

Tomato & Cucumber Slices

+

MAYO

Mayo

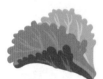

Chopped Romaine Hearts

+

Bleu Cheese Crumbles

+

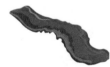

Bacon Bits

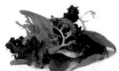

Mixed Field Greens

topped with

Shredded Cheese & Ground Beef

I would bring these in separate containers and combine at lunch.

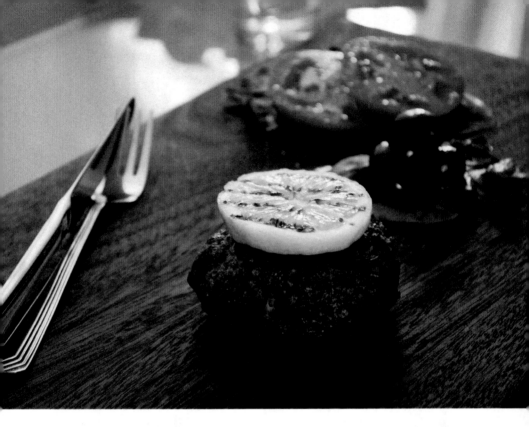

Burger patty warmed up and topped with all your
normal fixins... minus the bun and ketchup.

B.L.T.

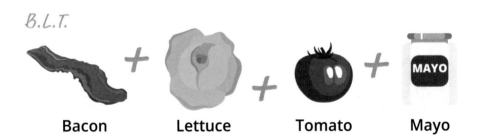

Bacon + **Lettuce** + **Tomato** + **Mayo**

Large tomato slices as bread with bacon and mayo.

Could also use lettuce as bread for bacon, tomato and mayo.

Crab Salad Lettuce Wrap

 *mixed with* + *served on*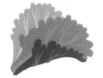

Chopped Crab Meat

Mayo & Celery

Lettuce Leaves

Egg Salad Lettuce Wrap

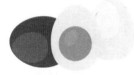 *mixed with* + *served on*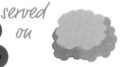

Hard-Boiled Eggs

Mayo & Chopped Green Olives

Lettuce Leaves

 + *served between*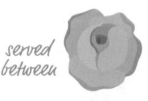

Sliced Ham

Swiss Cheese

Lettuce Leaves

Or serve it as finger food.

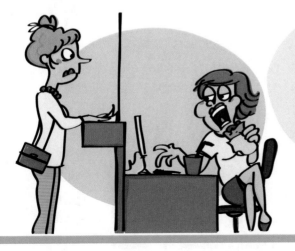

Mark my words... lettuce wraps are going to take the world by storm.

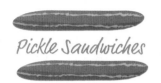

Pickle Sandwiches

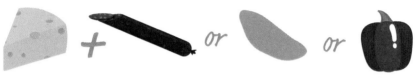

These work best with flat pickle slices cut long called "stackers" or "sandwich slices".

You can add anything to the slices to make a pickle sandwich, but here are my favs.

Cheese + **Uncured Salami** *or* **Bologna** *or* **Roasted Red Pepper**

MAYO

Ham Cubes

Ham Salad

Chicken Salad

Mayo + **Chicken Cubes**

Roast Beef + **Horse-radish**

Deli Ham Slices *rolled up with* **American Cheese Slices** *dipped in* **Mayo and/or Mustard**

A squirt of mayo in the center before roll up is good as well.

Can trade out mayo for yellow mustard and any cheese you prefer.

Riced Cauliflower (frozen) *stirred up with* **Cheddar Cheese** *placed on* **A Bed of Lettuce**

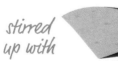

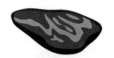 +   rolled up with

Roast Beef + **Horseradish Sauce** *rolled up with* **Cheddar Cheese Slices**

 *warmed up & dipped in* or or

Pre-Made Meatballs **Sour Cream, Mayo or Horseradish**

Fun Fact: All hot dogs are pre-cooked.

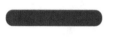 +

Uncured Hot Dogs **Bag of Frozen Veggies**

Like I said in the breakfast section, if you are too busy, rushed and impatient for real food, it's still good to grab something quick...

A keto or low carb friendly meal bar or shake can work great for lunch if you're in a pinch!

 or

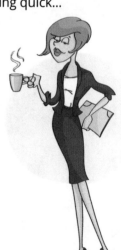

Meal Bar **Shake**

My favorite brands are Premier Protein & 310.

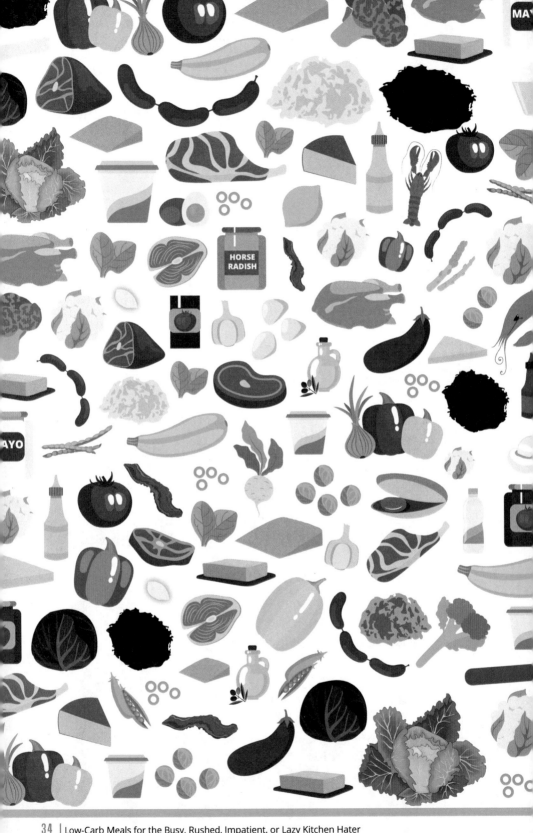

CHAPTER 4
Dinner Options
or Dinner Systems

STOP THINKing about the plate method. It just made everything worse. Fill your plate with veggies and protein. Drink water. Health solved.

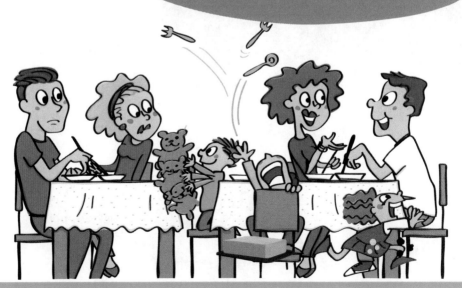

*Remember when going out to dinner **used** to be the easy option?*

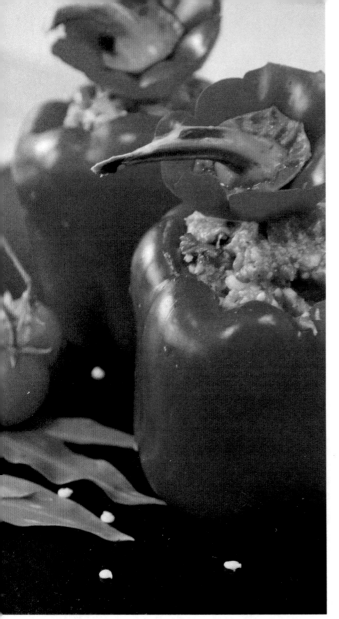

Stuffed Peppers

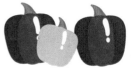

Peppers

stuffed with

**Ground Beef,
Chopped Onions
& Peppers**

or

Tomatoes

*Place in baking dish &
bake for 1.5 hours
at 350 degrees*

*I make about 6
at a time.*

Stuffed Zucchini Boats

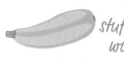

stuffed with

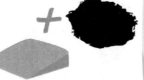

Zucchini

**Cheese &
Ground Beef**

*Bake at 1 hour
at 350 degrees
(6 boats)
reduce cook time
for fewer boats.*

Cordon Bleu

Cheese Stick *rolled up in a* **Slice of Ham** *placed in a* **Chicken Breast**

Roll up 1 cheese stick in a slice of ham

Place this in a chicken breast that has been sliced down the middle (don't cut it in half)

Bake for 45 minutes at 350

 Broccoli Florets *mixed with* 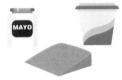 **Mayo, Cheese & Sour Cream**

Mix well and bake for 1.5 hours at 350

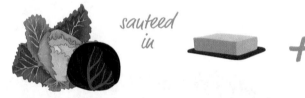 **Pre-Shredded Cabbage** *sauteed in* **Butter** + **Ground Beef**

Sauerkraut

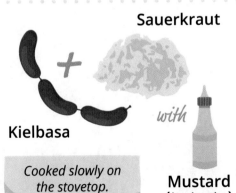 **Kielbasa** +

with **Mustard (to taste)**

Cooked slowly on the stovetop.

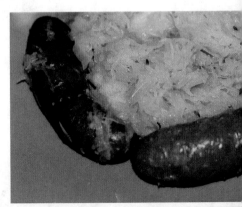

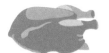 **Chicken**
 Tomatoes

 Spinach

> This is good for the slow cooker.
>
> Add chicken to cooker on high for an hour.
>
> Start to break it apart and add tomatoes and spinach.
>
> Cover and cook on low.
>
> Eat when you remember.

  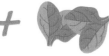

Stuffed Pork Chops **Spinach (Fresh or Frozen)**

> If frozen, make sure it's drained or it's a runny mess.

  Ricotta

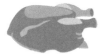 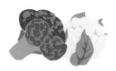

Chicken Breast **Baked Broccoli & Cauliflower**

> Throw it together in a baking dish.

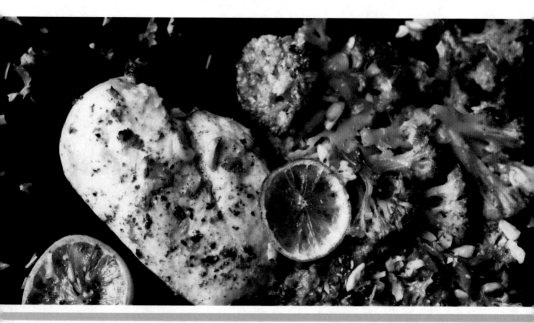

Riced Cauliflower Recipes

Save Time & Energy! Get Riced Cauliflower from the frozen section.

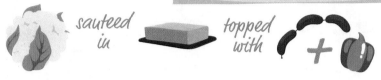

Riced Cauliflower *sauteed in* **Butter** *topped with* **Sausage Slices & Green Peppers**

Cook peppers & sausage separate. Then put on top of cooked cauliflower.

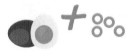

Lobster Meat *cooked with* **Riced Cauliflower** + **Gouda**

I think Gouda stinks, but it's your call. Cheddar worked just as well.

Fried Riced Cauliflower

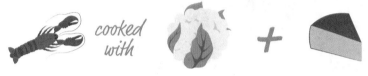

Riced Cauliflower *mixed with* **Egg & Chives**

Just like fried rice, add egg directly to the riced cauliflower in the pan and sauté.

Add chives once heated through.

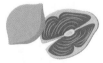 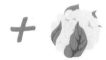 

Lime Salmon + **Cauliflower Rice**

Pan Baked Sausage & Green Beans with a side of Cauliflower Rice.

Salmon on the stovetop with lime... that's it.

Cook Cauliflower rice with butter & seasoning.

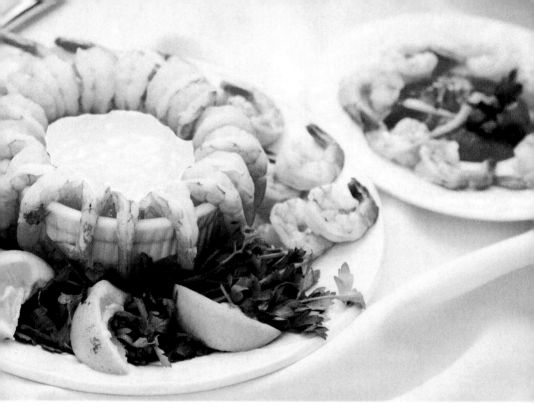

Shrimp Cocktail

 dipped in 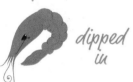 +

Shrimp

Horseradish & Mayo

A little bit of horseradish goes a long way.

Stovetop shrimp is my favorite and easiest.

 wrapped in with a side of 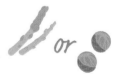 or

Scallops

Bacon

Asparagus or Brussel Sprouts

Hold bacon in place with a toothpick.

Put scallops in broiler for 10-15 minutes, but keep checking.

This is best broiled. If you don't know where your broiler is, Google it.

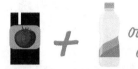 + **on top of a**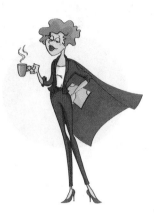

Tomato Paste   **Heavy Cream**   **Burger Patty**

This was a super power I stumbled upon.

Add ⅛ cup tomato paste with 1 cup heavy cream and cook on the stovetop. It's awesome and you can put in on top of anything.

 topped with

Eggplant Slices   **Mix of Ham & Parmesan**

Fry both sides of eggplant on stovetop.

Then add topping.

 baked with +

Cauliflower   **Hot Sauce**   **Mozzarella Cheese**

This is where I step it up a bit and get 2 dishes dirty.

Mix cauliflower pieces in bowl with hot sauce and cheese.

Spread in baking pan and cover. Bake at 350 degrees for about 45 minutes (until soft).

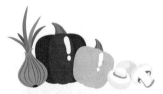 **with or without**

Fried Onions, Peppers, and Mushrooms   **Tomato Sauce**

Can also put this on top of riced cauliflower.

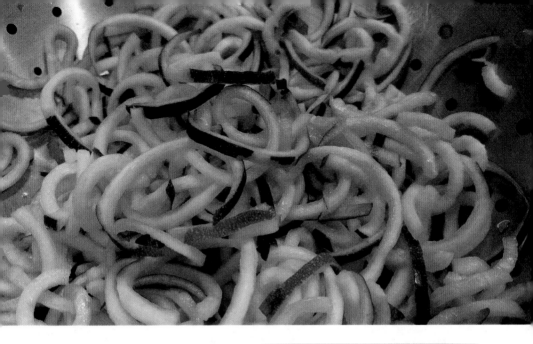

 Mussels

cooked in

 Tomato Sauce

served over

 Zoodles (Zucchini Noodles)

You need a tool to make these. OR guess what? Zoodles are also in the frozen section now.

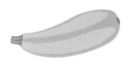 **Zoodles (Zucchini Noodles)**

+ 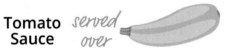 **Garlic**

+ **Parmesan**

+ **Olive Oil**

 Corned Beef

on top of

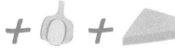 **Sauerkraut**

topped with

 Sour Cream

Corned beef comes canned or deli (go with deli). *Think Reuben.*

+

Sautéed Broccoli Raab   **Chopped Tomatoes**   *on top of*   **Cooked Pork Chop**

You can overcook pork chop but I eat it anyway.

To prevent though... or at least try... keep it covered while it cooks.

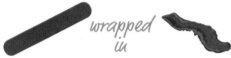

wrapped in

Uncured Hot Dogs   **Bacon**

Broil in oven.

Side of yellow mustard as dipping sauce.

I hear shaved brussels sprouts from a food processor cooks quicker... but then I would have to clean the food processor.

 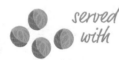 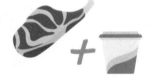

served with

Sautéed Brussel Sprout Halves   **Cubed Pork Chop**   +   **Sour Cream**

 + +

Mashed Turnips   **Garlic**   **Butter**

Boil the turnips (or get canned, since turnips take forever to boil through and you are super rushed).

Drain well since they are super watery and then mash.

Cabbage Leaves

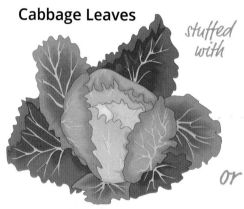

stuffed with

Ground Beef

Spinach

or

Ground Turkey

+

Cheese

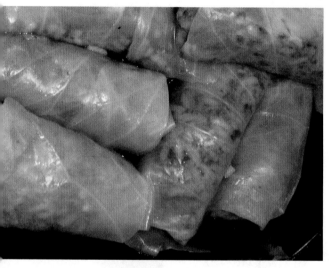

You need to boil the cabbage leaf first a bit (5 minutes each) so they are pliable.

Make the meat and veggie or cheese mixture in a separate bowl and spoon onto leaves.

Roll together (toothpicks help).

Sautéed Cabbage (cut sideways to get strips)

Sausage Slices

Green Pepper

topped with

Boiled Cabbage

Butter

Salt & Pepper

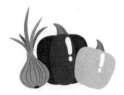 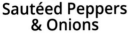 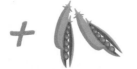

Sautéed Peppers & Onions + **Snap Peas** *add optional* **Cubed Steak**

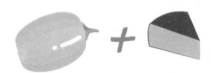

fried in **Green Beans** **Butter** + **Steak**

> I can't make a steak to save my life, so bribe a family member to cook this and focus on the green beans.

> This is a Sunday only recipe.
>
> Bake the entire squash in oven for an hour but make sure it's cut in half (400 degrees).
>
> Scoop out the guts and mix with sauce and cheese.
>
> Fry it on the stovetop.

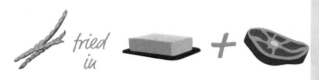

Twice Baked Spaghetti Squash **Sauce & Cheese**

I know after dinner you will want something sweet and I'm sure you've noticed that there is not a dessert section. That is intentional. Not because you will not eat dessert ever again, and NOT because there are no recipes.

It's because, dessert usually requires mixing, pouring, beating, folding, greasing or whipping. And remember, I'm busy, rushed, impatient and hate the kitchen. Dessert requires more effort.

If I need something sweet, I grab a chocolate square with 70% or above cocoa...aka dark chocolate. I can easily unwrap a piece of chocolate.

Besides, I'm trying to stop the sweet habit.

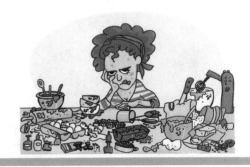

CHAPTER 5
Stuff I Do on Sunday

Sunday is a universal (almost) day of relaxing. Well, it's supposed to be; in reality it's when we try to play catch-up or try to get ahead for the week. Don't pretend this is not true. If I am on the ball, I would prep meals for the whole week. I'm usually not. So, instead of pretending I'm perfect, I focus on the tasks that will give me the MOST stress if they are not done. Those are also the tasks that sabotage my good intentions to eat proper food.

So, I need you to ask yourself. *What meal during the week do I most often give in to EASY instead of healthy?*

THAT is the meal you plan and prep for on Sunday. That is usually dinner. We have a weird tendency to want something different for dinner everyday, but are ok with the same breakfast and lunch week after week. Notice that? Pick the problem meal and focus on that first on Sunday. Remember, it's only effort until it's a habit.

The other habit I would highly recommend is having a family dinner. We really like to step up our game for Sunday dinner and get the whole family involved. This means it's a better quality meal with more love stuffed in than we will get the whole week. If you think that doesnt matter you're wrong. Did you ever notice how food tastes awesome when someone else cooks it; someone who loves us? That is the secret ingredient. That is why my mother's fried eggs taste sooo much better than mine. They are made with love.

I also think you should try making a Sunday Salad (if it's summer) or a Sunday Soup (if it's winter). This is something you can eat and pick at all day, and it takes very little time. Yes, even soup. Our schedules are different on the weekends and therefore our meals are off too. That's ok, but it gives us a lot of chances to de-rail from our goals. If you go to a church service, start the soup as soon as you get home. If you don't attend church, start the soup mid-morning. It will be ready to eat in an hour and get even tastier throughout the day.

Here is my soup recipe. Remember, I am the queen of busy, rushed and impatient, and I can make this without a recipe in front of me.

Wrinkle Soup

1. Look in the fridge for wrinkled or wilting veggies and chop them up *(or bribe a family member)*.

2. BEST soup veggies: onions, chopped carrots, celery, sliced cabbage, chopped peppers

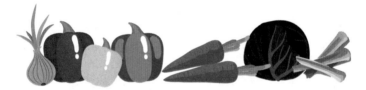

3. Add a stick of butter to the bottom of a soup pot and melt.

4. Add chopped veggies to bottom and saute until soft or brown... or you remember frantically that they are cooking.

5. Add spices like garlic salt, italian seasoning, salt and pepper. Don't get crazy, you can add more later.

6. Add broth OR the cheap easy way is to add water and bouillon cubes.

7. Bring to a boil and then simmer.

8. As it is simering you can add a meat if you like... I cheat and add rotisserie chicken.

9. DON'T ADD UNCOOKED MEAT TO SOUP if you want to eat it in an hour.

10. SOUP IS ON!

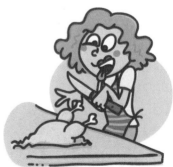

Here is another easy one:

1. Get a Crock Pot or Soup Pot.

2. Look in the fridge for wrinkled or wilting veggies and chop them up *(or bribe a family member)*.

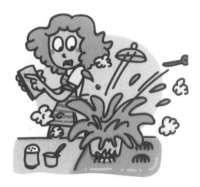

3. BEST soup veggies: onions, chopped carrots, celery, sliced cabbage, chopped peppers.

4. Add a stick of butter to the bottom of a soup pot and melt.

5. Add chopped veggies to bottom and saute until soft or brown.

6. Add 1 can of tomato sauce and 1 can of diced tomatoes.

7. Fill up with water.

8. Let simmer slowly and enjoy once flavors have combined.

9. I always need to add salt.

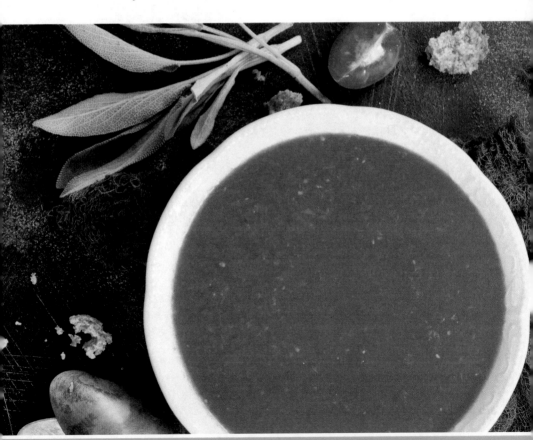

The Other Things I Tend to Focus on for Sunday

Make sure we have clean clothes...

at least clean underwear. Nothing induces a scramble more quickly than realizing you have no clean clothes. It is frowned upon to exit the house naked these days, so please check everyone's underwear drawer at the very least. Find the socks.

Make sure the shoes are accounted for and double check the keys are hung up before you go to sleep on Sunday night. Everything else can likely be de-wrinkled in the dryer and misted over with febreze to get through until Monday night when you can do at least one load of wash.

Check the stock of food staples for the week...

Quickest way to eat the wrong thing is to not have the right thing on hand. I know I know. I cannot stand the crowded lines the weekend creates at the grocery stores, but most stores are open very early. Some stores are open all night.

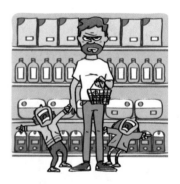

If you can, get up early and enjoy a quiet and peaceful shopping experience with a hot cup of coffee. I did this with my first kid who used to get up obnoxiously early, but then continued after I realized how much easier it made my life.

A few words for a heads up. The deli is closed early and there may be fewer check outs open as well.

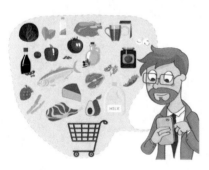

The other option, is to take advantage of stores that offer ordering online and curb side pick up. This is a life changer. You avoid all the unnecessary but very tempting purchases you would otherwise make, and you can keep your jammie bottoms on. Since I am busy, I always missed out on the best pick up times, so I had to go in anyway. Either option is kinda nice.

Take a nap...

Seriously. By Friday, you are dragging because you started the week off in a sleep deprivation. I like to put on the football game, if it's fall, and pass out on the couch for an hour. True story.

Make sure prescriptions, dry cleaning, pet food, bank deposits and random school or work errands are done before Monday... if possible.

WHY? Every single store has a snack section full of candy at checkout. Each trip is like running a gauntlet. Get it all done in one day while your will is strong and before the stress of the week weakens your resolve.

Since I am excellent at anticipating human actions, here is a bonus section for you.

Low-Carb Foods to Go

What Can You Take Along So You Won't be Tempted to BUY the King Size M&M?

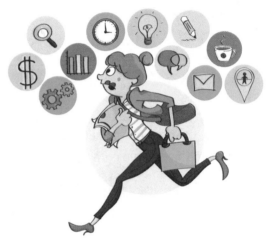

The biggest temptation to start going carb-crazy is when you're out and about, and that hangry feeling hits.

You have no snacks in the car or on your person, to sustain you. You even forgot the sparkling water and the coffee thermos *(or open coffee mug if you roll like me)* you lovingly packed.

The Burger King or Dunkin Donuts drive thru window beckons enticingly. The cafeteria at work is serving quesadillas with chocolate cake for dessert. It's all so tempting and it seems a bit intentional. As if the universe is asking you if you REALLLY want to eat properly. The answer is yes, but you have to be ready.

Instead of falling prey to the temptation of convenience foods, get into the habit of being just as sneaky as the lunch lady by stocking up on your snack options and having them ready to take on the go. This will keep your fuel tank reasonably filled while you're out at work, running errands, or just driving from here to there trying to accomplish what you need to. It also helps while you are bored and trying to convince yourself that you can stop at one Oreo.

ONE Oreo! That is as ridiculous as ONE potato chip.

What to Buy

Lunch Box

Soft, wipeable fabric and vinyl-lined is best
(mine has mermaids... don't you dare judge me).

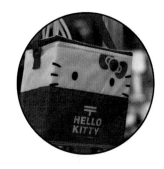

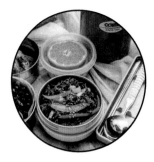

Storage Containers

Small ones with tight-fitting, snap-on lids will minimize mess, but since I'm impatient, I get the best Ziploc bags the world has to offer.

Remember the commercial showing the Ziploc bag turned upside down with pasta sauce... that one.

Plastic Forks, Spoons, Napkins and Cups

Keep them in the car. Mine if full of McDonald's napkins from my days in denial.

I keep some in them glove compartment, so I can easily reach over and feed my face in the parking lot of whatever store made me the hungriest.

MAKE sure you have this double full during the holidays. Trust me!

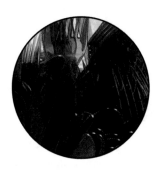

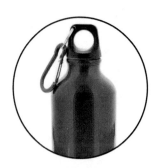

A Reusable, Aluminum Water Bottle

Prevent unnecessary trips to the soda machine or drink counter.

Full disclosure, I have a 12 pack of sparkling water in the trunk of my car almost all the time. The only time you have to be careful is when it is really cold and the cans can freeze and explode.

During the colder months, I leave the 12 pack in the front closet... behind the coats... in disguise.

I hate when people steal my sparkling road water.

What Foods to Stock

Eggs

Anyone who's told you that this way of
eating contains eggs and high-fat meats isn't
exaggerating... BUT it's your choice whether you
decide to eat these on repeat mode, or brand out to other options. Get
into the habit of boiling and storing a pot of eggs so you can grab a few
each day to stash in your food bag before you head out the door.

Mixed nuts and seeds. Not all nuts are created equal, carb-wise. The
higher the healthy fat count, the better. You can safely enjoy almonds,
macadamias, brazil nuts, sesame seeds, sunflower seeds, pumpkin
seeds, walnuts, pecans and coconut, among others. I tend to avoid
peanuts as they go down way too easy and soon the jar is gone. Cashews
are really high in carbs, but much better than a donut. In a pinch, any nut
is better than most other choices.

Avocadoes

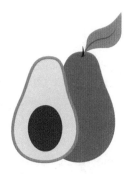

Avocado is an amazingly delicious and versatile
source of omega 6 fats that is low-carb friendly and
can be added or served as a side with many dishes.
The more you can diversify your fats (as opposed to
just eating tons of butter and cheese), the better for
your long-term health and success on this diet. You
don't have to create guacamole to enjoy avocados.
I typically throw one...ok two..into the lunch bag and
break it apart with my hands when I'm ready. You
can do that with a ripe avocado.

Canned Fish

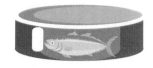

If you're a fan of tuna and salmon salads, you're
in luck. Fatty fish is one of the best choices for
your main source of protein at meal or snack
time when on a low-carbohydrate mission.
Just be aware that you should keep it to a few
servings per week until us humans figure out the mercury risk. Sardines
are the healthiest fish you can find, so if you enjoy those, you can keep
your pantry stocked with a variety of sardine selections to take along with
you in your lunch box. If that grosses you out, you are in good company.
I have tried so many times to incorporate these health jewels into my
routine and just cannot do it. *(Sugarless gum might be a good thing to have
if you'd like to avoid post-lunch tuna breath.)*

High-Fat Dairy
with the exception of milk which is high sugar... yes, even skim milk.

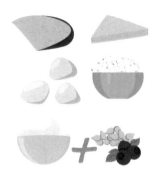

This includes cheeses of all kinds, including aged such as cheddar or Parmesan; soft cheeses such as brie and camembert which are higher in fat content; mozzarella and ricotta which are not aged; cottage cheese, cream cheese, sour cream, and full-fat Greek yogurt. I cannot eat greek yogurt without something, so bring along some nuts to add or a few blueberries.

Fattier Cuts of Meat

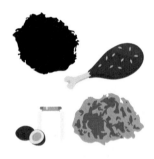

If you purchase ground beef at the store, try to select 80/20 or even 90/10. Poultry such as chicken or turkey is served best when it's higher-fat cuts of meat such as leg or thigh. If you do buy meat that's a lower fat content, you should supplement the meal with an additional source of fat - for example, cooking with olive or coconut oil, or serving your meats with mayonnaise or a mayo-based dip.

Keep in mind, from a common sense perspective, what it would take to remove fat from a food that contains fat naturally. *GROSS!*

Fiber-Rich Green Vegetables

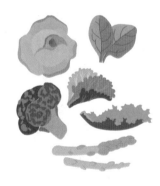

Just writing that makes me vomit in my mouth a little as my mind flashes back to the days as a child... trying to choke down spinach. Trust me, you taste buds change. I can eat spinach now, I just don't like saying it out loud. PLEASE Avoid carrots, corn, yellow and orange squash, and potatoes of any kind as much as possible. If you need to know the worst of the worst... it's corn. No Corn.

Leafy greens like romaine lettuce, spinach, kale, chard, celery, collards and broccoli are amazingly healthy. Turnips and cauliflower can be cooked and mashed as a potato alternative. Asparagus and peppers, too, are okay for low-carb eaters. Tomatoes and eggplant can be consumed in limited amounts if you are very strict. I don't eat either veggie everyday so I barely pay attention to this rule. However, you could be one of those people that eat tomatoes like apples, so I need you to be aware.

Reference List for Those that DON'T EAT Animal Products

The process is the same for those that don't eat animals.

The cooking oil will need to be avocado oil or even coconut oil. Add veggies, nuts & seeds together and enjoy. I prefer cooked veggies, but raw is amazing as well.

I know protein is always a problem, so here are the foods to include in larger quantities.

High Protein Seeds

Chia

Pumpkin

Hemp

Flax Seed

Sesame Seeds

Highest Protein Veggies

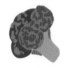

Broccoli

Avocado

Turnip Greens

Asparagus

Cauliflower

Okra

Brussels Sprouts

Arugula

Mushrooms

Pages for Your Creations

_____   _____

_____   _____

_____   _____

_____   _____

_____   _____

_____   _____

_____   _____

_____   _____

_____   _____

_____   _____

_____   _____

_____   _____

_____   _____

_____   _____

_____   _____

Acknowledgments

For my mother who taught me to make the best of what you have and showing me just how much that is.

For my family who endured hundreds of different food combinations over the year as my ability to create low-carb meals was under construction.

For my husband who never hesitated to gobble down my latest creation, taking each taste test in stride with a shrug of his shoulders.

For my patients and clients who had faith to make changes despite naysayers and critics.

For God, who instilled a continuously running motor in my brain and a desire in my heart to change lives for the better.

About the Author

Dr. Krista Ellow, PharmD., BCACP is a clinical pharmacist turned diabetes health coach who is on a mission to make the world of medications makes sense again! She is the host of her own podcast called, "The Angry Pharmacist" where she shares her experiences in the world of healthcare and the big misses that have occurred, particularly in the treatment and management of diabetes.

She has spoken on multiple podcasts herself, including Low-Carb Conversations, to talk on the exponential increase in the use of pharmaceuticals as the mismanagement of diabetes continues.

As a board certified expert in chronic disease, she spent years applying the traditional methods of diabetes management until her eyes were opened by a particularly stubborn patient; whom she continues to be grateful to. She realized that the medications she was using didn't make things better and didn't make patients healthier. They just changed the numbers on the lab sheet. This started a deep dive into the research surrounding diabetes best practices. What she found made her switch her entire approach, and now she uses food to help her patients heal, recover and overcome diabetes.

In this latest work, she shares her method of assembling meals with ease to transition people with high blood sugars into the world of low-carb living. She has used this eating style to prevent medication additions, elimination medication needs and reverse the prediabetes in both her and her sister among hundreds of personal clients. She shares her message of common sense diabetes eating with people encumbered by pills and injections with the bigger goal to change how this disease is treated on a large scale.